Introduction

How well one does in life is somewhat directly proportional to their physical and mental health. A body not in its best condition cannot be expected to give its best performance. It cannot give what it does not have hence can only operate within its conditioned capacity. To become the best version of oneself there has to be optimum mental and physical health. Great mental and physical health is a direct result of two major components which are, what one eats and physical fitness which comes about as a result of exercise. These are fundamental and foundational basics of life that cannot be overridden or compromised

Human nature makes us want to eat fancy food that may not necessarily be good for us. The fundamental approach to eating well for the sustenance of good health is by understanding what makes up the human body and also the food being consumed. Without that understanding eating habits become a case where one throws punches in the air and wins by chance or opportunity strikes. This approach is not sustainable and leaves the human body vulnerable to attacks. Knowledge and understanding of the body and what makes up the food being eaten is what will give constant and consistent healthy outcomes.

This write up aims to bring enlightenment or deeper understanding on the nature and origin of the human body and the food around us. The Creator concept is applied throughout this literature. The main idea over and above religious affiliation is to give understanding on the critical foundational aspects of health and wellness as a pre-requisite to one achieving their highest good or becoming the best version of themselves; be you a Hindu, Jewish, Islam, Christian, atheist or any other religion. You are not excluded. A body remains a body irrespective of your religious inclination. The same basic principles apply to anyone and everyone.

How do I Cynthia Arumero the author know all this? I am an open minded and all encompassing Christian. Throughout the years I have realised that we were created to depend on each other and one can benefit from other people irrespective of their beliefs, background or religious affiliation. Before religious affiliation life is a basic to everyone. We can benefit from each other if we approach things with open minds. Once upon a time I was a hard-liner Christian and am still a Christian. I would not hear anything about taking medication from hospitals let alone herbs. I had been erroneously indoctrinated to believe that prayer only should heal me and if I do not heal it means I have not prayed well or hard enough.

I had a major turning point in my life whereby fortunately or unfortunately I fell ill to the point of death. I prayed and got prayed for but could not get quite healed. Unknown to me, the Creator or the Universe had begun taking me through a learning and healing process. This process has taught and revealed to me the wholeness and divinity of nature and my relationship with it as well as how I can use nature to become the best version of myself. It has been eleven years from the period of illness to the point of writing this literature. I have physically healed, got mindset transformation,

trained as a herbalist and gained significant experience
and understanding of what makes me up and my life
continues to level up as I get to know more and apply
the knowledge to my personal life. I therefore, now seek
to share this healing, knowledge, experience and
understanding with all mankind irrespective of who they
are or where they come from in this publication.

One of life's basic facts and principles is, you can only
manage and control what you know and understand. One
of the mandatory basics of education worldwide should
have been an understanding of the human body and its
relationship with nature ahead of anything else. There
really isn't much sense in learning or teaching people
how to run and manage the world when they do not
understand or know how to manage themselves.

The writing of this literature is my testimony as I
transition into my higher self and ultimately into
greatness. Before I fell ill, before I understood and
applied what I share in this literature, before I recovered,
I could not see myself being able to write a book,
becoming financially independent and running my own
things, not depending on a job for survival but this is
where I am and looking to greater and mightier things
all single handed.

Chapter 1

Human body basics..........

In the story of creation we gather that man was formed using the earth or soil then the Creator breathed His spirit into man and man became a living being. (*Genesis 2:7....and Jehovah God went on to form man out off dust from the ground and to blow into his nostrils the breath of life and then man became a living person - New International version bible*). The Creator installed regenerative, reproduction and repair wisdom or instructions in people, plants and animals. Since then people, plants and animals multiply through reproduction and they self regenerate, heal and repair as and when necessary.

Body self regeneration happens when body cells die and new cells are created to replace the dead ones. *(The National Institute of General Medical Sciences explains: Regeneration as the process of replacing or restoring damaged or missing cells, tissues, organs and even entire body parts to full function www.nigms.nih.gov/education/fact-sheets/Pages/regeneration.aspx*). Every second that ticks the body generates millions and millions of new cells to replace old, dysfunctional or dead cells. In the same manner that skin cells die and peel off, cells inside the body also die and are washed off and out of the body as waste. This means that the body is always undergoing a constant and consistent process of self regeneration and recreation. Every now and then you have new body cells and a completely new body. These aspects of self reproduction, self regeneration and self repair ensured that the Creator did not have to keep recreating, regenerating or repairing injuries to living things. The body is auto-set to do that for itself.

Man is made of flesh and blood. Believe it or not, the substances that form the liver, the skin, the hair and the kidneys are minerals and elements found in the earth.(*Genesis 2:7....and Jehovah God went on to form man out off dust from the ground and to blow into his nostrils the breath of life and then man became a living person - New International version bible*). Their formula and combination is unique and known to the Creator or the Universe only and remains a mystery to man. The human body routinely and periodically regenerates and repairs itself using resources available to it within the body system. For instance, if one does not drink enough water to cleanse off dead cells and toxins as well as assist with the millions of internal body processes, the internal environment becomes contaminated and dehydrated. That same contaminated content is what the body uses to regenerate body cells when the need arises and that affects our well-being. Cell regeneration wisdom and instructions will not stop functioning because there are inadequate resources or contaminated environment. This means the quality of body cells, internal organs, skin and appearance is a direct reflection of the state of things inside the body- i.e. our internal body conditions. Man therefore has been given control, power and influence over how he turns out by what he chooses to take into his body.

Adequate intake of clean water and an internal environment with abundant resources for cell regeneration and repair ensures a faster regeneration or repair process which results in healthy body cells and ultimately a very efficient and effective body system. Such a clean and healthy environment results in overall quick healing in times of health attacks while an unclean internal body environment results in a slower or longer regeneration and healing process and a weak, less effective and inefficient body system.

If chronically ill or suffering from some form of ailment, take advantage of the process of the continuous regeneration process to feed nutritious and balanced diets into the system to provide the body with resources to regenerate a new body as the old affected cells die and are flushed out as waste. Through the regeneration process an entirely new healthy body can be made. It may take a while but with the right mindset, commitment and focus change is inevitable and it surely and certainly will come.

Likewise, when a plant does not have enough water its cells shrivel and this is evidenced by wilting. If the water situation around the plant does not improve, the plant eventually dries up and dies.

Humans and animals also go through a similar process. It sets off as a feeling of weakness then develops into lying down and not being able to move or carry out any activities and may even lead to hospitalisation. If the situation is not resolved, this may eventually lead to loss of life.

People who live in hot climates consume more water than those in cool or cold climates on a daily basis. Through sweating and perspiration, water is lost from the human body a lot faster and needs frequent replenishment. At any point and time the body should have a balance of the water it carries internally against the demands of its external environment.

In the same context as with water, the mineral and nutrient content within the body should also be enough to cope with the stress, weather, regeneration, repair and routine daily activities the body undergoes. When such a scenario exists, a state of wellness and well being prevails in a person. Absence of that balance initially sets off a craving which if not resolved then develops into discomfort or restlessness. This restlessness and discomfort if not addressed will further develop into body weakness and illness as the body resources continue to deplete.

Cell, tissue and organ deterioration and eventual damage due to failure to address the lack of resources required, deteriorates in phases. The situation develops from little simple to address and reversible damage, then to moderate damage which may take a bit of time to resolve and then further into a chronic situation where extensive damage may have occurred and will require more effort and dedication to resolve. Such cases are usually known as chronic illnesses. In worst case scenarios, the situation becomes unresolvable and the organ eventually stops functioning and may need an organ transplant. In cases where organ transplant is impossible it may eventually lead to death.

Failure of one internal organ to function can result in death because all body organs depend on each other for optimum performance. Internal organs are each other's bridges. They connect one part of the body's internal environment to another. If a bridge malfunctions, all internal organs are affected and if it completely breaks down a section of the body completely disconnects from the other. This cuts off supply of resources needed for the efficient function and survival of other organs leading to eventual shut down of the whole system.

The body has eleven major body systems that perform different functions. These systems are interdependent upon each other for functionality and effectiveness

The following systems and their functions were extracted from :
(https://images,app.goo.gl/G9qpvY31FPruZyKs5)

1. Nervous system
Coordinates the body's responses to changes in the internal and external environment.

2. Integumentary system
Temperature regulation, waste removal, sensory info and protection

3. Respiratory system
Delivers oxygen to the body and removes carbon dioxide

4. Excretory system
Rids the body of wastes, including excess water and salts

5. Digestive system
Converts food into smaller molecules that can be absorbed into the blood stream and transported to the rest of the body.

6. **Skeletal system**
Provides structure and support to the human body

7. **Muscular system**
Works with the skeletal and nervous system to produce movement, also helps to circulate blood through the human body

8. **Circulatory system**
Delivers oxygen and nutrients through blood to cells and different body parts through the blood

9. **Endocrine system**
Controls growth, development, metabolism and reproduction through the production and secretion of hormones

10. **Reproductive system**
Produces, matures, nourishes, and stores gametes for reproduction.

11. **Lymphatic (immune) system**
To remove pathogens and other infectious diseases from the human body.

External body organs rely on the well being and optimum functioning of the internal body system. It is possible for somebody not to have legs, hands or eyes but still be able to live normally using artificial systems around them to cope. The same cannot be said for the heart, liver, kidneys and all other internal organs. Malfunction or absolute dysfunction of any one of these will result in the whole system packing up and being sent back to mother earth 6 feet below the earth surface.

Exercise is a fundamental requirement for the proper functioning of the entire body system. It releases or activates necessary required energy by nutrients, body cells, tissues, organs etc for the transportation of required substances, speeding up of body processes. The more one exercises the more effective and efficient the body processes. Lack of exercise translates to the exact opposite. In addition to eating well, exercise has to come in. It would be like adding sugar to tea and not stirring the tea. the sugar will be there, not dissolved and will sit at the bottom of the cup. It will be very very sweet at the bottom and tasteless at the top. Stirring the tea dissolves the sugar and evenly distributes it into the tea. This is what exercise does for the body in relation to nutrients.

Chapter 2

Plant basics....

In order for us to fully comprehend the life of the body we live in, we have to understand the concept and the biological science behind plants. All plants retrieve nutrients from the earth or soil to use together with other atmospheric components like carbon dioxide and sunlight for their growth, survival and reproduction. The Royal Horticultural Society explains this process as follows *(Plants need a range of mineral nutrients to be able to function and grow.*
Plants absorb nutrients from the soil through their roots, then move them up through the stem.
*https://www.rhs.org.uk/advice/understanding-plants/how-plants-absorb-nutrients.)*Each plant has its own set of wisdom or instructions which makes it unique and different from other plants. The uniqueness is visibly evident in the size of the plant, the shape and colour of the leaves,the fruits and the plant's life span.

An orchard can have a variety of trees i.e. a guava tree, lemon tree, avocado tree, mango tree, peach tree or any fruit tree growing in the same environment. Likewise a vegetable garden can also have tomato plants, potato plants, spinach, carrots, cabbages, kale, covo, egg plants, leeks, onions etc all growing under the same weather conditions, same soil structure, texture and earth minerals, elements and components yet they will produce different fruits and vegetables which will mature for consumption in different seasons. This is because each plant carries in it wisdom and instructions to retrieve particular minerals and nutrients in particular quantities and combinations from the same earth and process them over a certain specified period of time to then produce a particular fruit or vegetable in a particular specific season.

The plant system through its roots retrieves or absorbs nutrients and minerals then transport them up the stem to the branches and leaves which then process food for the plant processes enabling them to produce unique fruits and vegetables guided by the naturally installed wisdom or instructions. The Royal Horticultural Society explains *this process as follows (Plants need a range of mineral nutrients to be able to function and grow.*
Plants absorb nutrients from the soil through their roots, then move them up through the stem.
https://www.rhs.org.uk/advice/understanding-
*plants/how-plants-absorb-nutrients.)*In simple terms the same mineral elements and nutrients are used by different plants in different combinations to bring out the different outcomes in the form of fruits and vegetables.

Fruit trees and vegetables produce seed either carried inside the fruit or in a pod or some protective casing. The seed contains wisdom and instructions which, when planted, subjected or exposed to conducive conditions bring forth another plant of the same type.

Why do different fruits or plants carry varying quantities of seeds? This is Creation or Creator order and a clear message and direction that the plant fruits, leaves etc should be consumed, replanted and reproduced at a rate equivalent or directly proportional to the number of seeds the fruit or the plant carries. Why else would the Creator put more seeds in one plant and less in another?

Different plants have different life spans. The plants with shorter life spans generally carry more seed while those with longer life spans carry moderate amounts of seed with some fruits like avocado, apricots and plums carrying only one seed. These variations in lifespan and seed content indicate the rate or frequency at which the plant leaves or fruit should be consumed and seeds replanted for reproduction.
Trees are bigger and taller in size with longer life spans while vegetables are generally smaller and shorter with shorter life spans. Trees take years to mature and bear fruit and can live for decades and even centuries in some instances for example the baobab tree. The baobab fruit carries a significantly large amount of seed compared to other fruit trees. The fruit and its leaves are highly nutritious and filled with loads of vitamins. This is a typical example of a tree whose products should be taken in large quantities because of their nutritional value and should also multiply to cater for high human nutritional demands.

Vegetable plants generally carry more seed for reproduction while trees carry less seed. They usually mature in 90 days or more depending on type of vegetable and its life cycle. Some vegetable plants are seasonal while others are not. Seeds can be planted for reproduction at the end of their life cycle.

Low lying plants tend to have more seed because they are also largely consumed by animals that creep, crawl and walk the ground. Animals like rabbits, goats, sheep etc may not be able to climb up trees but can access the low lying plants. The abundance of seed in such plants is to cater for the high demand from both people and animals. There should be reproduction of such plants in volumes in direct proportion to the seed content. As plant height increases some living things are excluded from consumption of those plants because of height disadvantage. Such plants tend to have seeds for reproduction in moderation.

When a fruit is in formation, it feeds off nutrients from the leaves of the plant. Orange tree leaves will give the same benefits that oranges give because whatever is contained in an orange comes from the leaves. The leaves also contain the instructions and nutrient combinations that give oranges their colour and they release to the fruit the nutrients for the process. Fruits contain easily and readily digestible nutrients and sugars.

Leaves contain the same nutrients in slightly more complex forms such that they have to be taken through a process of breaking down complex nutrient structures so that the become soluble. They are usually steeped in boiled or very hot water to breakdown the complex structures so that they become soluble and are taken as teas. The tender or new leaves of a tree are thinner, lighter in colour and the nutrients in them are more soluble and easily retrieved.

The older the leaves grow the more food is stored in them and the more complex the nutrient structures. They become thicker and darker in colour as a sign of the richer food stocks. The nutrients are less soluble and the leaves need to be boiled to break the complex structures into substances that are easily digested and absorbed by the human body. They are usually taken up as teas or strong concoction.

The barks, stems and roots of the plants will also carry even more complex structures of the same substances found in the fruits and leaves because they also serve as nutrient storage sites.

The leaves of a plant also known as the kitchen of the plant is where plant food is made. The University of Illinois Extension explains the process as follows : *Leaves are the site of the food making process called photosynthesis: in this process, carbon dioxide and water in the presence of chlorophyll(the green pigment) and light energy are changed into glucose(a sugar). This energy rich sugar is the source of food used by most plants. https://web.extension.illinois.edu/gpe/case1/* When leaves are shed off or eaten or taken off by other living things for whatever reason the plant would be expected to die. Seasons will wipe out all leaves from a tree and leave absolutely nothing but the tree will still not die. After cutting off a large part of a tree, it will bud and grow again as long as the roots are alive underground. All this happens because whenever there is a deficiency on the plant the stem and roots release the nutrients stored in them for the leaf regeneration process and any other processes the plant needs to carry out. These stored nutrients are broken down by the plant into simpler structures for the use of the plant by small protein substances called enzymes. They are then released into other parts of the plant based on the same wisdom and instructions that specifies the unique combination of minerals, elements and nutrients.

Having understood this, we see that the whole plant from the root to its tip contains the same nutrients in

varying complexities. It can therefore be concluded that
in the absence of fruits and leaves people can still
benefit from the roots, bark and stems of plants. These
however have to be boiled longer than leaves are boiled
so that the complex structures in them are broken down
to release nutrients stored in them into forms that are
easy to digest, easy to absorb and use by the human
body system. The nutrients stored in barks, stems and
roots are however more concentrated since they are
storage sites.

Chapter 3

The Critical Link of Life .....

Having gone through the basics of the human body and the concept and science behind plants we will now explore the link between plants, animals and humans.

The relationship between man and plants is that the fruit trees and vegetable plants through their leaves, fruits, stems, bark etc directly replenish the body system of required or depleted substances. How does that happen? As discussed earlier plant natural wisdom makes it take up from the earth certain or particular minerals in unique proportions and combinations that then result in the formation of a particular fruit unique to that particular plant. That combination of minerals, elements, nutrients and salts is carried in the fruit, leaves and rest of the plant. On eating that fruit or vegetable all its resource wealth is released into the body's systems and enriches the body with its contents. This release supplies the body cells and organs with the resources needed for body cells and body parts regeneration in the body self renewal process and continuous day to day healthy

functioning according to daily activities and weather
conditions. At this juncture it should now begin to add
up why people take fruits or vegetable broth to someone
who is sick in hospital.

The roots, stems and barks of the plant also contain
same nutrients as fruits and leaves but in more
concentrated forms as discussed earlier. Their
consumption should therefore not be at the same rate as
that of fruits and leaves. Unlike fruits they are not sweet
and do not have a pleasant taste. In most cases they are
bitter. The concentrated versions of nutrients stored in
roots, stems and barks also have capacity to address or
cure some conditions and ailments in humans that low
concentrations in fruits and leaves may not be able to
rapidly address.

Each second that passes, a zillion chemical processes
take place all over the whole body. Body processes grow
the body, repair or heal, regenerate, digest, remove dead
cells, toxins, absorb nutrients, create energy etc for use
by cells as they carry out body processes and for other
internal and external practical body activities such as
working, walking, talking, seeing, hearing, cooking,
thinking, laughing etc. Body cells use nutrients, minerals,
vitamins, water etc to make all these things happen. For
the liver to function at its best it requires certain
minerals, vitamins and nutrients in certain quantities or
proportions and combinations. The same applies to the
kidneys, the heart, the spleen, the brain etc. Each body
part has its own specific combination of minerals,
nutrients and vitamins required for it to operate at its
optimum capacity as naturally required by the body.
These are requirements are in two categories i.e. for self
regeneration as old cells die and new ones made and for
its efficient and effective functioning. Body
requirements vary according to gender, age, body weight,

height and daily activities. A pregnant woman will demand more nutrients and minerals as compared to one who isn't. This is because she is creating another being. She needs enough calcium to form all the 256 bones that form the skeletal system among other things. A man who does a lot of exercising, working out or hard physical work will demand some substances more than one who sits at his desk and works using his brain. Their nutritional demands vary based on factors such as those.

Weather conditions and external environment also exert their own pressure and influence the rate at which the body uses up nutrients and minerals in the body. If living under hot weather conditions where a lot of sweating takes place as the body tries to cool itself, salts are lost through the sweating process.
Any compromise in the quantities of minerals, nutrients and vitamins required by any body organ to function efficiently and effectively will result in that organ not operating at the required level and that in turn will affect the other body organs and the body system as a whole. For instance if the body does not have enough salts or sugars for the efficient functioning of the heart, the heart will not operate at its required capacity. A craving for salty or sweet food is set off. Meanwhile this means that not enough oxygen will reach all body parts and the body feels weak. The effective and efficient functioning of individual internal organs becomes affected and ultimately the whole body. Prolonged failure to address the issue may result in one experiencing fainting, shortness of breath and may need to be connected to an oxygen supply while the problem gets addressed.

Likewise excess nutrients, minerals and salts will result in toxicity of the environment the body organ is operating in. Too much of a good thing can become poisonous, leading to illness and even death. Salt gives flavour to the food, however too much of it makes the same food inedible and a danger to the body. The same applies with the sugar, oil, zinc and magnesium contents among other things required by the body. Excess of anything will affect the cells, organs and the body as a whole. It will also result in feelings of discomfort and un-wellness and if not addressed could result in illness and ultimately death. We have seen this with high blood sugar. The body however has Creator installed wisdom, instructions and mechanisms to remove any excess substances and maintain the correct balance of nutrients, minerals and vitamins it requires at any point to function effectively.

As emphasized earlier a state of well being is achieved when there are adequate amounts of minerals, nutrients, water content etc for optimum functioning of body organs according to their individual requirements and ultimately the body as a whole. This is why nowadays upon visiting a medical facility for treatment they initially run blood and other biological lab tests to check for blood content and isolate or identify the the root causes of un-wellness and assist in prescribing the appropriate treatment for the body to be restored to normal function and wellness.

For one to maintain consistency in well-being there should be constant and consistent replenishment of required substances lost through breathing, eating drinking and exercising. NHS Health Scotland explains that: (*a well balanced diet provides the energy you need to keep active throughout the day and the nutrients you need for growth and repair, helping you to stay strong and healthy and help to prevent illness such as cancers https://www.nhsinform.scot/healthy-living/food-and-nutrition/eating-well/health-benefits-of-eating-well/*). The body cells and organs use whatever is taken in for

their processes and reject what they no longer require. If a required resource is missing the body places a demand through a craving. The National Geographic Society explains (*Food as one of the basic necessities of life which contains nutrients-substances essential for the growth, repair and maintenance of body tissues and for the regulation of vital processes.*
https://education.nationalgeographic.org/resource/food/
.)

The Creator through His wisdom also created seasons and along with those seasons vegetables and fruits to replenish the body of lost or needed nutrients to cope with the demands and stresses that arise due to weather conditions, normal daily activities or unique seasonal activities or conditions. It is by design that a particular tree will yield a particular fruit in a particular season. The reason being that, the tree has been divinely programmed to take up from the earth or soil certain combinations and proportions of minerals, water and nutritional elements; process them over a particular period before presenting them to mankind as attractive and delicious fruits.

Mineral salts, nutrients and vitamin deficiencies can also arise as a result of off season's activities and weather conditions which would have used up resources needed by the body to cope with current season's demands.

Besides being seasonal, plants are also geographical and climatically influenced. Creator has set up earth such that certain plants are found in certain geographic areas depending on the climatic or weather conditions. A baobab tree is very prominent in areas with high temperatures and almost non existent in cool climates. This has to do with the particular nutrient needs and requirements of the people living in those climate conditions. In some cases you will find variations of the same plant family growing under different weather conditions for example sweet apple or graviola or soursop in West Africa is the equivalent of custard apple in southern Africa. There are some plants that will thrive under any conditions but may taste different depending on the environment they developed under.

Water melons for instance are seasonally available. They are a summer fruit where temperatures are high. They are known as hydrating fruits because they have high water content which when consumed replenishes the body's water levels. Lycopene the red pigment or colour in water melons protects the body against damage caused by pesticides, herbicides etc which are largely used in summer as it is the planting season due to the availability of rains. Its also an antioxidant which protects the body from damage caused by free radicals hence protecting against cancer. Lycopene improves heart health and prevents against sunburn. The nutritional value of Lycopene specifically targets the well being of the heart. The proper or efficient function of the heart ensures blood is pumped to the whole body so that nutrients, water and oxygen reach all parts of the body. People are usually very active and up and about in summer which places a higher demand on the heart's function.

Additionally the number of seeds in a fruit is a direct indication of how much of it to consume in any given season. More seeds mean more of that fruit should be consumed, moderate number indicates moderate consumption while one seed means regular eating. One should aim to eat all the fruits available in a season according to the seed content prescribed frequencies. Every fruit has its own major unique role which other fruits may not satisfy.

Each fruit and each plant almost always contains a certain amount of all required nutrients by the body. They however carry dominant nutrients and give the fruit or vegetable its dominant function. This effectively means each plant has dominant or main functions and secondary functions. It also further means that functions and benefits from fruits and vegetables never exist in isolation. The other present nutrients and elements still provide their benefits to the body even in their lesser quantities. These will however not be adequate to meet the body's demands or requirements of the particular substance and problems caused by deficiencies of such substances will still manifest though not in a devastating way. That is why it is therefore necessary to consume all fruits and vegetables available in a season. It is natural and normal to like or favour a certain fruit or vegetable over another. Too much of one thing though will not be good or healthy for the body.

It is important to note that a craving is different from a liking of a particular fruit or vegetable. A craving comes unexpectedly and creates a desire to consume a particular thing which is then quenched by eventually consuming that particular thing which one may not ordinarily like, while liking is having an interest to eat a particular thing because it is pleasant. Liking makes one buy a thing even when they did not really feel hungry or a burning desire to consume it.

The body requirements, if correctly, adequately and timeously replenished to meet demand would age healthy, youthful and graceful. Youthfulness in appearance and agility can be maintained even in old age. Mental and physical agility is very possible but requires discipline.

Cells have a lifespan. They age,die and are replaced. In an article written for the Scientific American by Mark Fischetti and Jen Christiansen, they expand on regeneration process through findings by other scientists and explain that: *The human body replaces its own cells regularly. Scientists at the Weizmann Institute of Science in Rehovot, Israel, have finally pinned down the speed and extent of this "turnover." About a third of our body mass is fluid outside of our cells, such as plasma, plus solids, such as the calcium scaffolding of bones. The remaining two thirds is made up of roughly 30 trillion human cells. About 72 percent of those, by mass, are fat and muscle, which last an average of 12 to 50 years, respectively. But we have far more, tiny cells in our blood, which live only three to 120 days, and lining our gut, which typically live less than a week. Those two groups therefore make up the giant majority of the turnover. About 330 billion cells are replaced daily, equivalent to about 1 percent of all our cells. In 80 to 100 days, 30 trillion will have replenished—the equivalent of a new you.*
https://www.scientificamerican.com/article/our-bodies-replace-billions-of-cells-every-day/. Creator instilled instructions for replacement never change. They remain the same. The only difference is that organs grow bigger in size and consequently the whole body. The skin wrinkles, sagging and wasting as we see externally is also an indication of what is happening to the organs inside. This is a direct consequence of the contents of the blood and lack of physical exercise. The regeneration process can only use what it has in activated form and it produces results directly proportional to what is available. So the wasting of the body is basically due to inadequate or lack of required resources to uphold and maintain the growing size. For instance, if we give a 7 year old child a full orange we cannot expect that same one orange to cater for the

needs of a 20 year old, 30 year old, 50, 70 year old body and so on but we unconsciously continue to make our bodies rely on that one orange way after it has multiplied in size and age. This is one fact and factor human minds have failed to recognise and address. As the body grows there should be a corresponding increase of the intake of fruits and vegetables among other plant matter.

If plants retrieve nutrients from the earth or soil and can supply the body with everything needed then how does meat from animals fit into the picture? Animals eat the leaves and fruits of plants. They eat the unprocessed leaves and have digestive systems that process and reprocess the difficult to digest leaves and plant parts till they are soluble and can be absorbed into their blood stream and body system. Cows for instance have four stomach chambers and they chew the curd meaning processed food will come back by reverse peristalsis, gets processed again and goes back into the stomachs until it gets fully reprocessed and can be absorbed by their body system.

The nutrients from the digested food are absorbed into the blood stream and transported to all the body cells and parts of the animal. We have all witnessed very healthy looking cows, goats, zebras etc that feed on just plant matter. Some make a very captivating and pleasant sight. Animals like humans also process and store in their bodies what is contained in the plants and build up healthy, fleshy organs with shiny attractive skins. People then slaughter these animals and consume their juicy, tasty and fleshy meat. The meat is very healthy and contains nutrients beneficial to the human body. This then leaves the argument that people eat meat as a main protein source. Goats, sheep, cows, zebras and many other herbivores do not consume meat but still develop healthy, fleshy tasty organs from consuming plants.

It has always been recommended to consume animals that eat plants i.e. herbivores against animals that consume other animals i.e. carnivores. When a carnivore eats a herbivore then a person eats the carnivore, the person is now third in the nutrient benefit chain. Original nutrients were processed and absorbed by the herbivore meaning it would have used up the nutrients it absorbed from the plant food. The carnivorous animal therefore benefits more from eating the herbivore. This then compromises the benefits that can be accrued by a person through eating a carnivorous animal.

Chapter 4

Understanding the full nature cycle....

Animals, plants and humans are subsystems of one big natural ecosystem. They all belong to, relate and depend on each other in one way or another. One cannot exist without the other. All nature is made up of nutrients from the earth or soil and on dying or disposal it gets buried back into the ground or earth where it decomposes and disintegrates into the original small little individual nutrients. Upon disintegrating they enrich the earth or soil with nutrients they carried in them initially absorbed from the ground. These are then be re-absorbed by plants as organic matter. They are a ready source of high nutritional value and content needed by the plant and they make the plant grow into a very healthy plant.

Let us explore the process of setting up a compost. It involves loading up layers of dead, dry plant material such as branches and leaves, then adding a layer of soil and more dead plant material and remains from food stuffs, kitchen waste like egg shells, banana peels, chicken feathers, meat that has gone bad, potato peels etc and add another layer of soil on top. The number of layers depends on one's personal preference or interest depending on what they want to achieve. It may also be influenced by possible availability of soil and kitchen waste, garden waste, weeds, dead plant material etc. Some people actually sell compost. After a while all those things that were being added to the compost totally disintegrate and can no longer be separately identified. They all looks the same as soil except with a richer texture. The same happens when animals or humans die. They rot and disintegrate into their initial small particles and re-unite with the rest of the soil or earth. After a while everything looks just like the soil. Upon taking that enriched soil where some stuff which used to be living matter has disintegrated and adding it onto the ground where a living plant is growing, there will be a boost in the plant growth and healthy appearance.

Animal waste on the other hand is also plant material that has been processed by the animal in its digestive system and removed from the body for varying reasons such as being indigestible or excess and no longer required in the body. Though it is waste it still contains some of the elements, minerals etc that were initially extracted from the earth. Likewise if added to a plant or soil around a plant, it results in a boost in growth and the health of the plant. That is why animal waste is good manure or food for plants. It is a ready source of nutrients.

The reason why dead plant and animal matter and waste causes a boost or positive change in the growth and appearance of a plant is because nutrients that the roots would ordinarily grow in search of either along the ground or deep into the ground would have been supplied through the dead matter and waste. It becomes readily available.

Ever wondered why plant roots bend, twist and turn into different directions giving them varying unique shapes? This happens as the roots develop and grow in the direction in which the nutrients or water the plant needs and seek are in abundance. This behaviour is similar to that of a craving in a human being or animal. Plants have an inbuilt mechanism that makes them grow towards where what they require is. A part of a root my become thicker than one before it or after it, because at the point where it became thick, there was an abundance of resources it required that boosted its development. If the plant roots do not find required nutrients signs of poor growth and ill health begin to manifest in the shoot of the plant.In a lesson given by Haripriya Munipalli and Amanda Robb on https://study.com/learn/lesson/tropism-in-plants.html. They explain this process as *Root tropisms(turning) are important responses in plants allowing them to adapt to their growth direction. Tropisms are plant responses defined as directional growth responses to the directional stimuli. The movement of plants and their growth responses are categorized as plant tropisms. The movement in plant parts aids them in acquiring food, water, light, and nutrients for their growth.* The shoot is the part of the plant that is above the ground.

When a woman is pregnant, she has unique food cravings which arise due to a demand by the growing foetus in her womb. Satisfying the food cravings ensures required nutrients reach the foetus for a healthy development.

Bones do not easily disintegrate like flesh does. However after millions and millions of years upon continuous addition of soil on bones, pressure and temperatures increase upon them underground, they eventually disintegrate and convert to fossils from which fossil fuels are derived. When such a process takes place on dry ground coal and gas are formed and when it happens under the oceans or water bodies, petroleum products are are formed. These are for use by people and industrial activities. *NHS Health Scotland explains that a well balanced diet provides the energy you need to keep active throughout the day and the nutrients you need for growth and repair, helping you to stay strong and healthy and help to prevent illness such as cancers. https://www.nhsinform.scot/healthy-living/food-and-nutrition/eating-well/health-benefits-of-eating-well/* It can therefore be concluded that man, animals and plants are unique combinations of earth minerals, elements and components all retrieved from the earth or the ground and developed or brought together using Creator wisdom and instructions. They live and die and go back to the ground where they are reabsorbed by plants and processed into combinations that bring out edible leaves and fruits for animals and people. Trees also produce oxygen required by people and animals to live. In the absence of oxygen death becomes the status. People and animals release carbon dioxide which the plants need. Absence of carbon dioxide results in the death of plants. People, plants and animals are earth or soil expressed in unique ways as a result of unique mineral combinations and life is a continuous, interdependent, ongoing process and cycle of nutrients made up of the earth or soil, people, plants and animals.

Without knowledge and understanding of what constitutes the body, it is very difficult to successfully manage, maintain and uphold its well being. It either

gets damaged or destroyed and its life span
compromised from lack of knowledge. A concerted
effort to know one's body should be made, observe how
it reacts to certain things, listen to its demands, feel it,
understand it and take good care of it. Make an effort to
understand nature, relate and commune with it. If that is
diligently done then a long healthy life is assured.

Chapter 5

A reconciliation of facts

All plants have Creator given mandates. They release
oxygen needed by people and animals need for survival
as waste. They also absorb carbon dioxide a waste from
animals and humans and use it for its biological
processes. If carbon dioxide is not absorbed by the
plants, the air will become toxic and people and animals
will all die.

In addition to oxygen production each plant has its own
unique functions. Some have beautiful flowers that
decorate the earth, others give a pleasant smell, most of
them make delicious healing teas and they all provide
cools shades when its hot. Some produce fruit which is
food for both people and animals. Animals eat the leaves
of plants and at times the stems and roots too.

Eating the meat of an animal that has eaten the leaves of
a plant is not an evil or ungodly act. Eating fruit of a
plant is also not an evil or ungodly act. As explained in

earlier chapters the fruit actually develops using nutrients supplied through the roots and leaves of a plant.

Humans, plants and animals are dependent on each other for survival and form part of the cycle of nature. None of the components of the nature cycle is evil. Consumption of leaves, stems or roots and even flowers of a plant is in no way evil. They are all formed and develop using nutrients and elements from the earth or soil. If any of that should be considered evil,ungodly or unholy then it makes the soil or earth evil because all of nature is nutrients, elements and minerals coming from the earth and assembled in different and unique combinations to bring out the different things on earth. People, plants and animals are there for each other's well being using the earth or soil as a source of resources. It is a Creator designed natural survival ecosystem.

When one falls ill due to any of the reasons expressed above nature is the next best thing to heal them. If diet and nutrition are not well managed in relation to nature problems arise. If addressed early then they are easily surmountable. If left to deteriorate then hospitalisation will be the only way to go where higher level intensive treatment is administered.

Correct eating pattern or habit should be the first point of staying well and healing. Have you noticed that when a person is unwell they are largely fed on fruits and vegetable broth. Vegetable broth is made from different vegetables and almost always results in an unwell person regaining their appetite and energy. Against this background it is encouraged to love fruits, vegetables, spices, herbal teas in their varieties. Consume them in their seasons in appropriate quantities and you will maintain top notch health and may never have need to

take artificial medication for anything because this basically keeps sickness and disease away. *NHS Health Scotland explains that a well balanced diet provides the energy you need to keep active throughout the day and the nutrients you need for growth and repair, helping you to stay strong and healthy and help to prevent illness such as cancers.*
https://www.nhsinform.scot/healthy-living/food-and-nutrition/eating-well/health-benefits-of-eating-well/

There are beliefs among some religious sects that consuming herbs or leaves of plants is diabolic and a reflection of one's lack of faith, trust, not being very prayerful or weak belief in Creator and that Creator can heal just them.

Without foregoing the supernatural power of the Creator through prayer, it is evident that Creator already set up natural healing processes when He first created nature. It is by being responsible and taking good care of the body which is the temple of the Holy Ghost eating properly that maintains good health. A person cannot continue to be irresponsible and practice bad eating habits and continuously be praying and asking Creator just to heal them. It is not sustainable. Some sects believe that only water that has been prayed for heals. Water is just part of what the body needs. It does not have the capacity to address that which should be addressed by other minerals and nutrients from the earth. Water though effective has its limits.

It is therefore certainly not evil or diabolic to consume the leaves of plants as herbal teas or with cereals and meal porridge. If consuming a banana or a mango fruit is not evil then consuming mango or banana leaves cannot be evil either. From the first chapter we note that whatever is in a banana or mango actually came from the leaves and is found in the leaves and the rest of the plant too. In the same breath if it is not evil to consume the flesh or meat of an animal that ate leaves of a plant then it cannot be evil for a person to consume the same leaves directly.

The pharmaceutical industries have over the years understood the plant system and the healing nature of plants. Through chemical processes they conducted laboratory analyses of the constituents of plants to discover the dominant chemical structures and components that effect the healing aspect in plants. They then sought to replicate the plant systems process and started producing drugs en mass. They came up with systems of extracting nutrients and minerals from the earth and processing them in a laboratories and mass producing in factories. It is in a way similar to what a tree naturally does.

The major differences are that in the process of extracting the required substances and separating them from other unrequired substances from the soil, they use chemicals which may be harsh but still bring them to process a replica of the desired substance. Plants in contrast use pure naturally Creator installed wisdom, instructions and mechanisms and have a way of extracting the required elements from the earth and filtering out what is not required. Plants have a full combination and complement of minerals and nutrients while pills are largely usually made using the main active ingredient. An active ingredient is the identified dominant nutrient in a plant. For instance a moringa leaf can address many health issues. The same leaf can be processed to extract oil from it which can still address some health issues and the cake that is left after extracting the oil will also still be able to address health issues. This means the whole moringa leaf has components which can be separated and still be effective in their isolated versions. The isolated versions though can never be more powerful than the whole unprocessed moringa leaf. From this we can conclude it is better and more beneficial to maintain health by consuming various plant components as compared to then seeking healing from artificial.

Chapter 6

Healing and Healthy Lifestyles...

The Action Steps

Having learnt and understood the nature and cycle of life, let us now get into the different steps of how to maintain and sustain our beings. There is a table at the end of the book with benefits of fruits and leaves of plants. It is not exhaustive but simply a guide. An important fact to always bear in mind is that fruits become available in different seasons but the leaves of the fruit tree will be available in all seasons. In the absence of the fruit, the leaves will suffice.

Step 1
Self check your sensuality

Sensuality is a word derived from the word senses which describes the ability to sense things through Creator given sense organs i.e. nose, eyes, tongue, ears and skin or hands. Make it a periodic (weekly or monthly and after going through a sickness) ritual to check that your five senses are fully functional. Most people go through life without realising that some of their senses have packed up i.e. not functioning.

i)   Check if your taste buds still pick up the taste of food.

ii)   Do you still pick up smells even the faintest smell? Some people only pick up strong smells and some no smell at all. There are people who have taken bad smelly food and fallen sick when the smell of the food should have indicated to them its bad state and restrained them from consuming it.

iii) Do you still see clearly or you are now struggling with your eyesight?

iv)   Is your sense of hearing normal?

v)   Is your sense of feeling still intact? Some people can get scratched or hurt and not feel it. They may pick it up later and not be able to reconcile when and how they got hurt. You can touch your own feet, hands or any part of your body and check to see if you feel yourself.

vi)   Do you have an overall sense of well-being?

If there is something or anything wrong with any of the sensuality organs or aspect, it is a sure sign that something is no longer functioning properly, has packed up or is slowly packing. Sensuality was put in us for our own good. It gives the body messages and information for pleasure, protection and coordination among many other activities the body faces or needs to deal with. When sensuality is compromised or goes off the whole system is exposed and becomes vulnerable to danger.

Step 2
Detoxify the body

i)   The first daily detox ingredient is taking in adequate amount of water on a daily basis. Water provides a medium through which other nutrients can be transported into or out of the body system

ii)   Prepare and drink a blend of chlorophyll filled(green) vegetables and fruits. Chlorophyll the green colour in vegetables is a good detoxifying agent. Example : a blend of kale, spinach, cucumber, green apple, lettuce, broccoli, parsley, celery etc can cleanse the system at the same time enriching it with a burst of other nutrients.In an article written by Taylor Woosley on (https://www.fruityield.com/the-fruitful-life/chlorophyll-benefits-for-detox-more/. It states that: *infact, the most well known benefit of chlorophyll is its detoxifying properties, Studies have shown that chlorophyll promotes detoxification because of its ability to bind to heavy metals. Chlorophyll can also support health blood circulation and oxygen levels in the blood stream*)

iii) Garlic also detoxes the body and rids it of heavy toxins

Toxin overload in the body system can also cause mal or ineffective functioning of organs. It is usually a result of not taking enough water to help the body wash out unwanted elements causing them to stick or assimilate themselves in places where they are not wanted thereby making that place where they attached themselves face difficulties in functioning properly. There are fruits, vegetables, spices, herbs in the form of tree leaves etc that cleanse or clean up the body. Body detoxing process is very important and should be periodically carried out. Intensive detox should be carried out once a month and at most once in every three months. Unwanted material should not be allowed prolonged presence in the body system as it is an unnecessary, unhealthy and ailment causing overload.

Chronically ill people usually reach a stage where their medication ceases to be effective because their body system is overloaded with medications they have been taking for years. The solution to this is consistent and constant detoxing periodically. It relieves the body of the drug overload

Step 3
Replenish the body

Consuming all and every fruit in season should be a lifestyle. There are vegetables and fruits and plants unique to every season and these should be consistently and constantly consumed as fruit and vegetable salads. Make herbal tea blends from the leaves of fruit trees. These can be made by taking a few leaves off the plants and a few of another and steeping them together in boiled water then taking as a tea. Steeping works for tender leaves while older, thicker leaves should be slightly boiled. There is no limit to the number of leaves you can add but this should be approached in moderation starting with 3-4 leaves of each plant or as directed. As discussed earlier too much of a good thing can become poisonous. Fruits may be expensive but the leaves of the trees in the form of teas are an affordable alternative. The body self adjusts and restores itself to full functionality. It is important to note that no part of a fruit from its seed to its outer cover is useless. Each part of a fruit just like the whole plant from the roots, stems up to the leaves, flowers and fruits is useful. The outer shell of a coconut fruit, baobab fruit, avocado, melon, banana or orange peels, pineapples etc are rich with nutrients which can be extracted through boiling them. Throwing them away has been a gross misdoing.

The processes of system enrichment if continuously and consistently carried out may lead to eventual and complete healing even from the worst of ailments. Prevention is however better than cure.

Step 4
Keep a routine body maintenance schedule

i) Be observant of all the fruits and vegetables in season.
ii) Ensure that at least 3 times a week, make and take vegetable blends and/or fruit smoothies using a blender or alternatively eat fresh fruit or fresh vegetable salads. Aim to consume every fruit and every vegetable in season in each season.
iii) We discussed different geographical locations of trees. Drink herbal tea blends of trees and herbs in your geographical area.
iv) Drink at least two litres of water daily.

Step 5
Exercise Daily

i) Exercise for at least 10 - 15 minutes daily. Include a routine that shakes up the whole body like jumping jacks, jogging in one place, going up and down a flight of stairs or up and down a hill. Time yourself and increase distance as well as improve on exercising time.

When something is stationary it carries what we call potential energy. Potential from the meaning of the word potential means capacity to do something but not actually engaging in the act of doing it. You can consume good healthy food that gets transported to body organs by the pumping of the heart but when it gets where it should get, it sits there with its potential but not executing it. It accumulates and in the case of carbohydrates, further converts to fat. If a body engages in exercise, all body organs shake consequently shaking cells and their contents thereby converting potential energy into kinetic energy. When nutrients become kinetic they move and start releasing their power and potency into the body system and benefiting the body.

https://www.cdc.gov/physicalactivity/basics/pa-health/ *Regular physical activity is one of the most important things you can do for your health. Being physically active can improve your brain health, help manage weight, reduce the risk of disease, strengthen bones and muscles, and improve your ability to do everyday activities.*
Adults who sit less and do any amount of moderate-to-vigorous physical activity gain some health benefits. Only a few lifestyle choices have as large an impact on your health as physical activity.

Everyone can experience the health benefits of physical activity – age, abilities, ethnicity, shape, or size do not matter.

Chronically ill people who are on constant medication must also exercise on a daily basis. It helps with revitalising the system and bringing it to normal functionality and coupled with detox and good nutrition may lead to full recovery. Extracted from https://www.healthline.com/nutrition/19-benefits-of-exercise (*regular exercise has been shown to help boost energy levels and enhance your mood. It may also be associated with many other health benefits, including a reduced risk of chronic disease………exercise has been shown to improve your mood and decrease feelings of depression, anxiety and stress.)*

As expressed earlier not exercising is like adding sugar to tea and not stirring it. It remains undissolved and concentrated in one place while stirring gives the sugar energy, dissolves it and spreads it throughout the water sweetening the whole cup.

It is not enough to just eat well. Exercise **HAS** to be a part of it. One cannot be implemented without the other.

Extracted from
https://www.researchgate.net/figure/Medicinal-Plant-Uses_tbl1_298806992.

Plant	Detox	Benefits
Guava Fruit	anti-microbial and anti-fungal, anti inflammatory	Has high fibre which supports digestion, reduces menstrual and stomach cramps, heart health and regulates high blood pressure.
Guava leaves	Clears diarrhoea, reduces cholesterol, aids weight	Improves sperm count and fertility, Fight, relieves

	loss,manages sugar levels, fights cancer cells, clears acne, calms some fevers, anti-allergy	menopause symptoms, vaginal dryness, low libido, depression, fatigue, source of iron
Mango Fruit	anti-bacterial, anti-fungal, alkalise the body, balances cholesterol	Immune booster, anti cancer, anti-oxidant, rich in iron, aids digestion,
Mango Leaves	anti-inflammatory, balances blood sugar, stomach tonic	Helps with stomach ulcers, hiccups and throat problems, gall and kidney stones, cures respiratory issues, ear infections, heals burns, diabetes, hypoglycaemia, lower high blood pressure, relieves restlessness, voice loss,

		dysentery,
Avocado Fruit	anti-inflammatory	Introduces good cholesterol, eye health,skin health, heart health, regulates blood pressure, aids digestion, blood sugar health, cancer prevention, pregnancy health, bone health and liver health, brain health, arthritis, improves mood and mental health.
Avocado Leaves	natural toxin removal, anti-microbial action	hormonal balance, weight loss, skin and hair health, oxidative stress, protection from chronic disease and

		all the benefits under fruits
Avocado pit/seed	naturally removes any toxins	erectile dysfunction, Blood pressure, osteoporosis
Pumpkin Fruit	flushes out germs and toxins	enhances skin glow, improves digestion,mood enhancement, immune booster, heart health,muscle recovery, weight management
Pumpkin Leaves	anti-bacterial	improves blood production, improves bone and teeth health,maintains body tissues,dietary fibre, regulates testicular damage in men, sperm cell

		formation,pr otects the liver,cures anaemia and chronic fatigue, weight loss
Moringa Leaves	removes general toxins and arsenic toxins, anti-septic, anti-bacterial, anti-inflammatory	supports brain health,reduc es blood pressure, reduces blood sugar,lowers cholesterol, protects liver, improves lactation, high calcium content, weight and stomach health, prevents respiratory problems, brain health
Banana Fruit	cleans the gut and helps with bowel movement	instant energy source, powers the brain, reduces stress, cures heartburn,bo

		ne health,heart health, aids to sleeping, can soothe a hangover, prevent chronic diseases, calms muscles and prevents nerve impulses
Banana Leaves	anti-inflammatory	Immune booster, sore throat, blood dysentery, weight loss, high in anti-oxidants, reduces fever
Soursop/Graviola/Guyabano/Sweet apple Fruit	anti-bacterial, anti-inflammatory, anti-virul	cancer treatment, treats diabetes, addresses respiratory stress
Soursop/Graviola/Guyabano/Sweet apple Leaves	removes uric acid,anti-inflammatory,anti-bacterial,antimi	cancer treatment, treats diabetes, anti-oxidants,

| | crobial | treats gout, back pain, immune booster, helps with chronic ailments, gastrointestinal health, regulates bowel movement, relieves stress, depression and anxiety,hair health, eases respiratory stress,skin health, wound healing,heart health, fights fevers |
| Baobab Fruit | anti-inflammatory | rich in many important vitamins and minerals, weight loss, balances blood sugar,digestive health, immune booster |

Baobab Leaves		
Pawpaw Fruit	anti-inflammatory	Eye health, immune booster, rich in anti-oxidants, reduce cancer risks, heart health, chronic diseases prevention, digestive health and clears constipation, skin health, anti-aging
Pawpaw Leaves	Blood tonic/purifier	Diabetes or high blood sugar, treats urinary retention, fibroids, gastritis, all menstrual problems, .
Spinach	whole body detox, anti-inflammatory	cancer prevention, weight loss, boosts muscle strength, iron source, heart and

		cardiovascular health,fights cancer, lowers blood pressure, eye health, brain protection, supports bone health
Watermelon Fruit	removes uric acid and ammonia	Hydrating, regulates blood pressure, maintain electrolyte and acid balance, lowers risk of asthma, heart health and cardiovascular health, weight loss aid, skin hydration and health, provides collagen, good for pregnancy, kidney health because its a diuretic, aids liver

		functions, reduces possibility of cancer, eye health, rich in anti-oxidants
Watermelon Leaves	Immune booster	Supports heart
Hibiscus Leaves	Removes uric acid, liver fat, anti-bacterial	Supports liver, kidney, repairs digestive system, alleviates menstrual pain, restores hormonal balance

References

www.nigms.nih.gov/education/fact-sheets/Pages/regeneration.aspx

https://images,app.goo.gl/G9qpvY31FPruZyKs5

https://www.rhs.org.uk/advice/understanding-plants/how-plants-absorb-nutrients.

https://web.extension.illinois.edu/gpe/case1

https://www.nhsinform.scot/healthy-living/food-and-nutrition/eating-well/health-benefits-of-eating-well/

https://education.nationalgeographic.org/resource/food/.

https://www.scientificamerican.com/article/our-bodies-replace-billions-of-cells-every-day/.

https://study.com/learn/lesson/tropism-in-plants.html.

https://www.fruityield.com/the-fruitful-life/chlorophyll-benefits-for-detox-more/.

https://www.cdc.gov/physicalactivity/basics/pa-health/

https://www.healthline.com/nutrition/19-benefits-of-exercise

https://www.researchgate.net/figure/Medicinal-Plant-Uses_tbl1_298806992.